The Essential Acid Reflux Cookbook

Your Guide to Managing Acid Reflux

By

Heston Brown

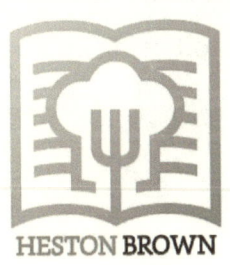

HESTON BROWN

Copyright 2019 Heston Brown

Thank you so much for buying my book! I want to give you a special gift!

Receive a special gift as a thank you for buying my book. Now you will be able to benefit from free and discounted book offers that are sent directly to your inbox every week.

To subscribe simply fill in the box below with your details and start reaping the rewards! A new deal will arrive every day and reminders will be sent so you never miss out. Fill in the box below to subscribe and get started!

https://heston-brown.getresponsepages.com

Subscribe
to our
newsletter

Your Email

Table of Contents

Chapter I - Smoothie Recipes for Acid Reflux

xxxxxxxxxxxxxxxxxxxxxxxxxxxxxxxxxxx

Recipe 1: Ginger and Banana Smoothie

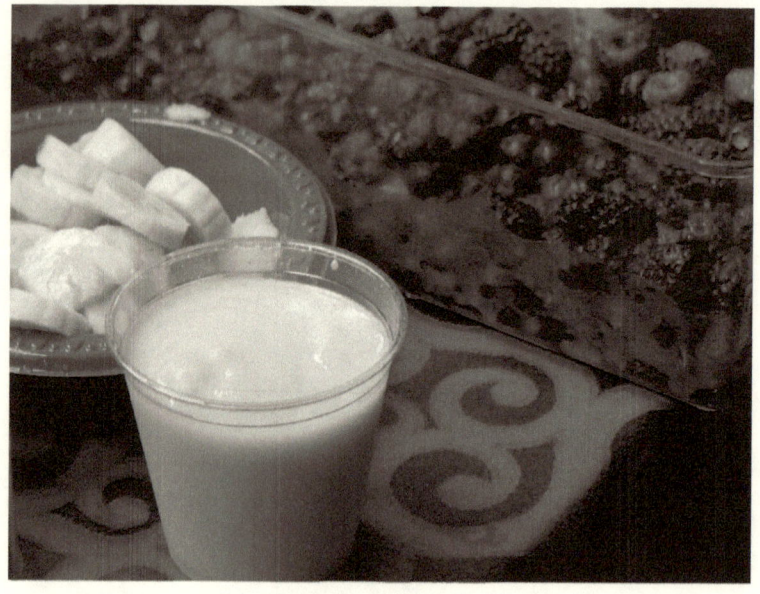

This smoothie is a great way to fight the acid that causes heartburn.

Yield: 1 to 2

Preparation Time: 10 to 15 minutes

List of Ingredients:

- 2 cups milk, low-fat
- 2 ripe bananas, peeled and sliced
- 1 cup yogurt
- ½ tsp. grated fresh ginger
- 1 cup plain yogurt, low-fat
- 2 Tbsp. honey

xxxxxxxxxxxxxxxxxxxxxxxxxxxxxxxxxxxx

Instructions:

Step 1: Place all the ingredients in a blender or food processor. Pulse until the ingredients are smooth and creamy.

Step 2: Pour the smoothie into 1 or 2 glasses and enjoy as soon as possible.

Recipe 2: Avocado and Strawberry Smoothie

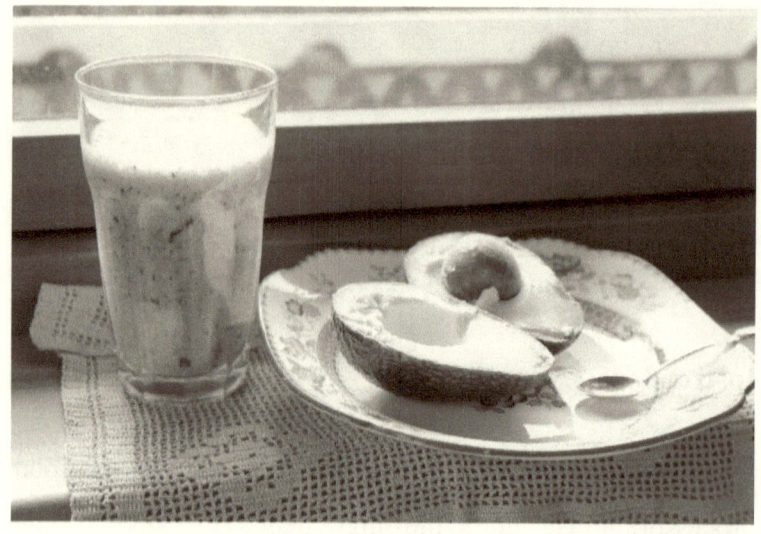

Smoothies make a great grab-and-go meal that won't aggravate acid reflux conditions.

Yield: 2

Preparation Time: 15 to 20 minutes

List of Ingredients:

- 1 avocado, skinned, pitted and diced
- 1/3 cup milk, low-fat
- 1 ½ cups sliced strawberries, frozen
- 1 Tbsp. honey

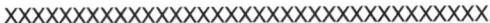

xxxxxxxxxxxxxxxxxxxxxxxxxxxxxxxxxxx

Instructions:

Step 1: Place all ingredients into a blender or food processor. Puree the ingredients until creamy and smooth.

Step 2: Transfer the smoothie between two glasses and serve immediately.

Recipe 3: Day on the Beach Smoothie

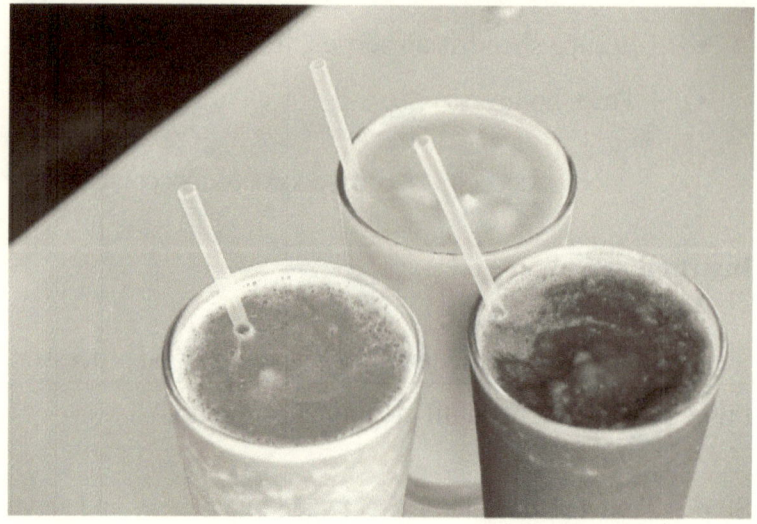

This low acid smoothie brings tropical flavors to the comfort of your own home.

Yield: 2

Preparation Time: 15 minutes

List of Ingredients:

- 1 cup mango, skinned, pitted and diced
- 1 cup pineapple chunks
- ½ frozen banana, peeled and diced
- 1 cup papaya, skinned and diced
- 1 cup almond milk or low-fat milk
- ½ cup ice cubes
- Fresh mint leaves, optional

xxxxxxxxxxxxxxxxxxxxxxxxxxxxxxxxxxx

Instructions:

Step 1: Place the mango, pineapple, banana, papaya, milk and ice cubes into a blender. Blend the ingredients until smooth.

Step 2: Pour the smoothie into 2 tall glasses. Garnish with fresh mint leaves.

Recipe 4: Red Beet Smoothie

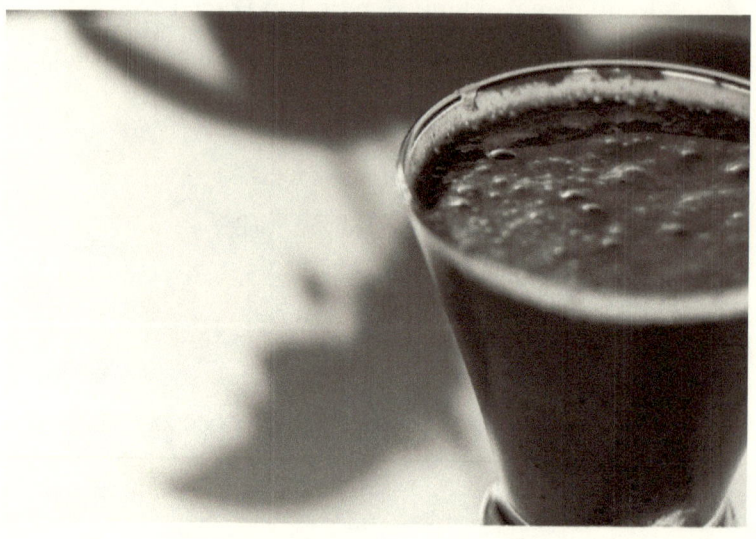

This mineral rich smoothie is great for suffers who want a delicious and cooling beverage without causing problems with their acid reflux.

Yield: 1

Preparation Time: 15 minutes

List of Ingredients:

- 1 cup red beets, steamed and peeled
- 1 cup kefir, plain
- 1 tsp. apple cider vinegar
- 1 Tbsp. honey
- Pinch ground cinnamon

xxxxxxxxxxxxxxxxxxxxxxxxxxxxxxxxxxxx

Instructions:

Step 1: Place all ingredients into a blender and blend until completely smooth.

Step 2: Pour the smoothie into a glass and enjoy immediately.

Recipe 5: Watermelon and Spinach Smoothie

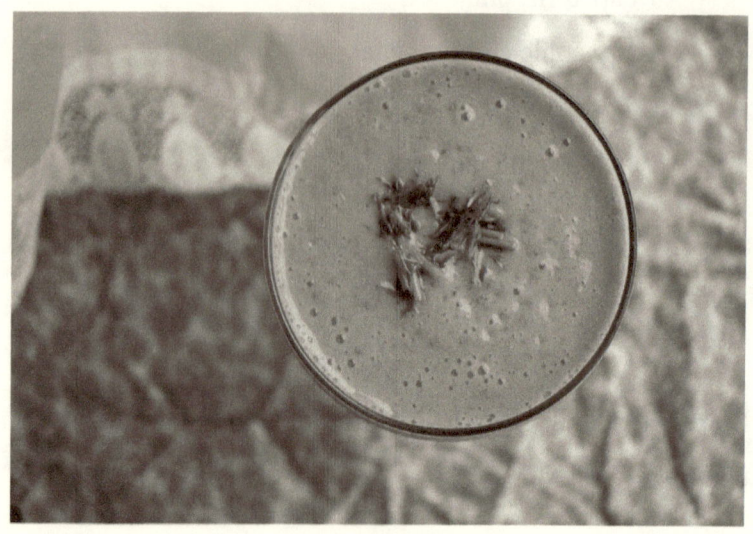

Who would have thought that watermelon and spinach could come together to create a delicious, low acid smoothie?!

Yield: 2

Preparation Time: 15 minutes

List of Ingredients:

- 4 cups cubed watermelons, peeled and seeds removed
- 1 cup baby spinach, fresh and destemmed
- 1 cup oats, soaked for an hour
- ¼ cup coconut, desiccated
- 1 cup ice cubes
- ¼ cup chopped walnuts

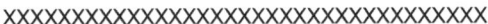

xxxxxxxxxxxxxxxxxxxxxxxxxxxxxxxxxxxx

Instructions:

Step 1: Place all ingredients into a blender and blend until the mixture is smooth and creamy.

Step 2: Divide the smoothie between two glasses and enjoy immediately.

Chapter II - Breakfast Recipes for Acid Reflux

xxxxxxxxxxxxxxxxxxxxxxxxxxxxxxxxxxxx

Recipe 6: Low Acid Pancakes

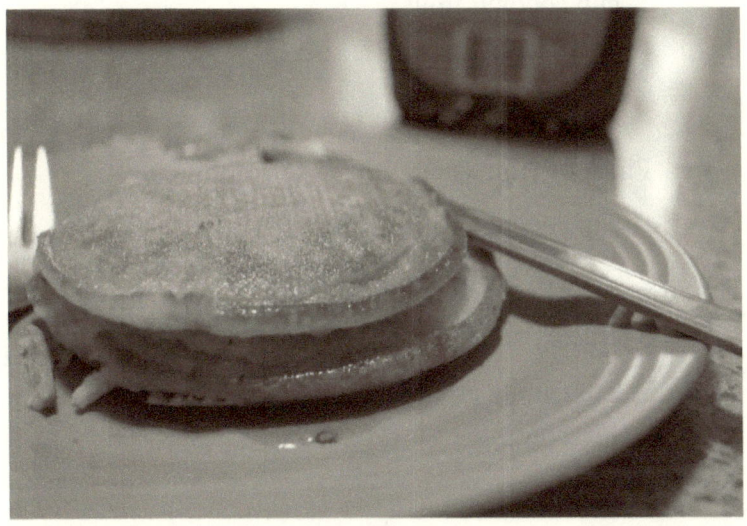

The addition of cinnamon gives these pancakes a nice flavor. For a complete breakfast, serve with your favorite fresh fruit.

Yield: 2

Preparation Time: 25 to 30 minutes

List of Ingredients:

- ½ cup coconut flour
- 1 Tbsp. cinnamon
- ¼ tsp. baking powder
- Pinch of Himalayan salt
- ½ cup coconut milk, no-fat
- 2 Tbsp. of coconut oil
- 3 large eggs
- ½ tsp. vanilla extract
- ½ Tbsp. honey
- Cooking spray

xxxxxxxxxxxxxxxxxxxxxxxxxxxxxxxxxxxx

Instructions:

Step 1: Place all the ingredients, except for the cooking spray, in a large mixing bowl. Mix the ingredients well until they are thoroughly combined. This is the pancake batter.

Step 2: Spray the bottom of a large skillet with cooking spray. Set the skillet on the stove over medium heat.

Step 3: Cook the batter from Step 1 as you normally would with any other pancake batter. Let the batter cook for about 3 minutes or until the bubbles begin to form. Next flip the pancake over and cook for an additional 3 minutes. Continue in this manner until there is no batter left.

Step 4: Serve the pancakes while still warm with your favorite topping.

Recipe 7: Breakfast Banana Bread

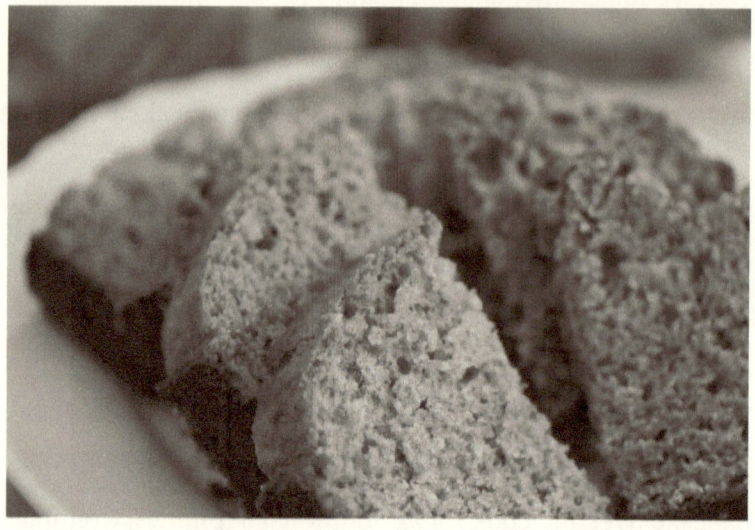

This banana bread recipe is a great grab and go breakfast meal that won't aggravate acid reflux.

Yield: 16

Preparation Time: 1 hour 25 minutes

List of Ingredients:

- 2 large egg yolks
- 5 large egg whites
- 1 1/3 cup sweetener, such as stevia or splenda
- 2 Tbsp. light spread
- 1 tsp. vanilla extract
- 4 bananas, peeled
- 1 ½ cups flour, whole-wheat
- 2 ½ cups flour, all-purpose
- 1 tsp. baking soda
- 4 tsp. baking powder
- ½ tsp. salt
- ½ tsp. nutmeg
- 1 tsp. cinnamon
- ½ cup wheat germ
- ½ cup buttermilk, non-fat
- 1 cup pecans
- 4 tsp. brown sugar, packed

xxxxxxxxxxxxxxxxxxxxxxxxxxxxxxxxxxxx

Instructions:

Step 1: Preheat the oven to 325-degrees. Use aluminum foil to line the bottom of a loaf pan. Set the loaf pan to the side for the moment.

Step 2: Add all egg yolks into a mixing bowl. Whisk for a few seconds. Add the spread and whisk again.

Step 3: Add the peeled bananas and mash into the egg yolk mixture. Whisk in the vanilla extract and sweetener.

Step 4: In a second mixing bowl, whisk the egg whites until they are frothy.

Step 5: In a third bowl, sift together both flours, baking soda, baking powder, salt, wheat germ, brown sugar, cinnamon and nutmeg. Add this mixture to the egg yolk mixture.

Step 6: Fold the egg yolk mixture into the egg white mixture. Carefully mix in the buttermilk before folding in the pecans.

Step 7: Pour the mixture into the prepared loaf pan from Step 1. Place the pan in the preheated oven and bake for about 50 to 60 minutes.

Step 8: Remove the bread from the oven and let cool. Turn the bread out from the pan and slice before serving.

Recipe 8: Quick Barley Breakfast

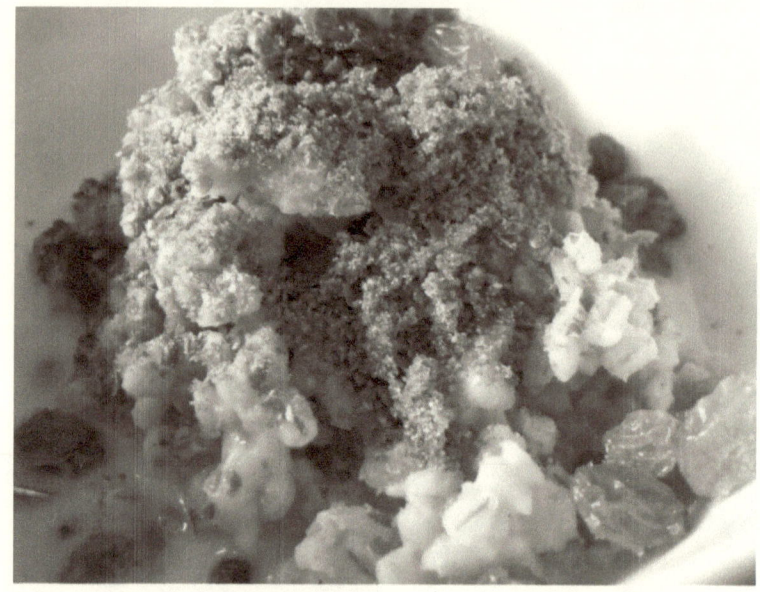

This quick breakfast can be prepared the day before so you can grab it and go the following morning without worrying about triggering your acid reflux.

Yield: 2

Preparation Time: 25 minutes

List of Ingredients:

- 2 Tbsp. honey
- 1/3 cup milk, low-fat
- ½ tsp. cinnamon
- 1 pear, cored, peeled and diced
- ¼ cup almonds, chopped
- 2 cups barley, cooked

xxxxxxxxxxxxxxxxxxxxxxxxxxxxxxxxxxxx

Instructions:

Step 1: Place the honey, milk, cinnamon and pear in a skillet. Place the skillet on the stove over medium-low heat. Let the mixture cook, while stirring continuously, for 10 minutes. The mixture should start to thicken a bit.

Step 2: Stir in the almonds and barley, and cook for 3 minutes.

Step 3: Divide the breakfast between 2 bowls and enjoy while still warm.

Recipe 9: Scrambled Eggs and Spinach

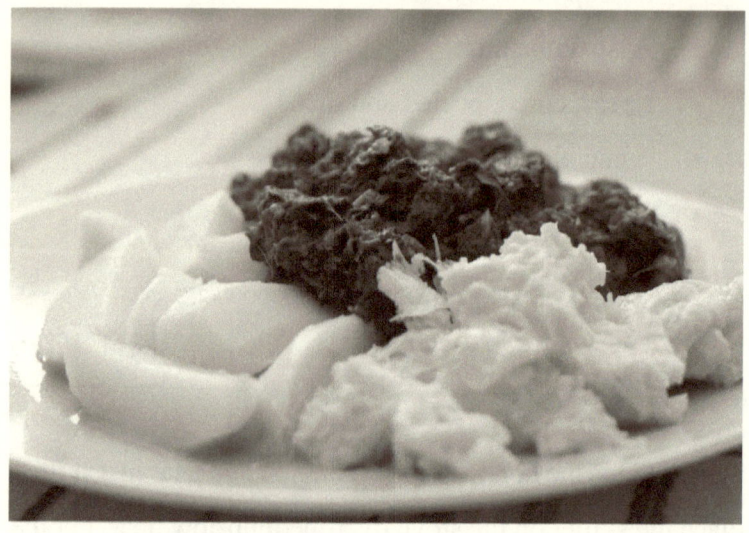

Not only is this breakfast recipe healthy and low in acid, it is also filled with protein that jump starts your day right.

Yield: 2

Preparation Time: 15 to 20 minutes

List of Ingredients:

- 6 large egg whites
- 2 large eggs
- 1 cup fresh baby spinach, finely chopped
- 1 cup ricotta cheese, low-fat
- Pinch salt
- Pinch parsley
- Cooking spray

xxxxxxxxxxxxxxxxxxxxxxxxxxxxxxxxxxxx

Instructions:

Step 1: Mix the egg whites, eggs and baby spinach together in a mixing bowl. Add the parsley and salt and beat lightly. Set the bowl to the side for the moment.

Step 2: Spray the bottom of a large skillet with cooking spray. Set the skillet on the stove over medium heat.

Step 3: Pour the egg mixture from Step 1 into the heated skillet and cook for about 4 to 5 minutes. Scramble the mixture while a spatula during the cooking process.

Step 4: Once the eggs are cooked through, divide them between 2 plates. Enjoy while still warm.

Recipe 10: Easy Peasy Oatmeal

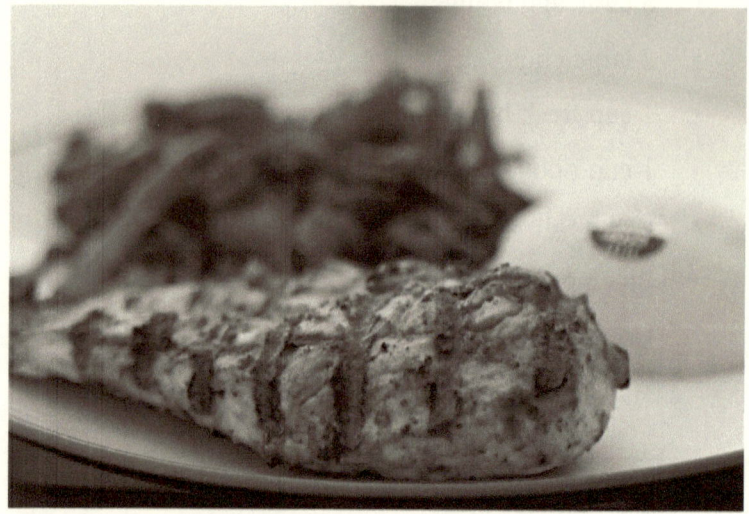

This easy to fix oatmeal recipe taste delicious and won't cause problems with your acid reflux.

Yield: 2

Preparation Time: 20 minutes

List of Ingredients:

- 1 cup oats, quick-cooking
- 1 cup water
- 1 cup milk, non-fat or almond
- Pinch of Himalayan salt
- Honey, to taste
- Ground cinnamon, optional

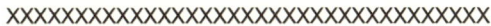

xxxxxxxxxxxxxxxxxxxxxxxxxxxxxxxxxxxxx

Instructions:

Step 1: Cook the oats as directed on the package. After about 3 minutes, turn the on medium low and add 1 cup of water.

Step 2: Stir in the remaining ingredients and let cook for about 8 minutes. The liquid should be absorbed.

Step 3: Divide the oatmeal between two serving bowls. Sprinkle the top with ground cinnamon, if desired, before serving.

Chapter III - Lunch Recipes for Acid Reflux

xxxxxxxxxxxxxxxxxxxxxxxxxxxxxxxxxxxxxx

Recipe 11: Grilled Chicken with Spinach

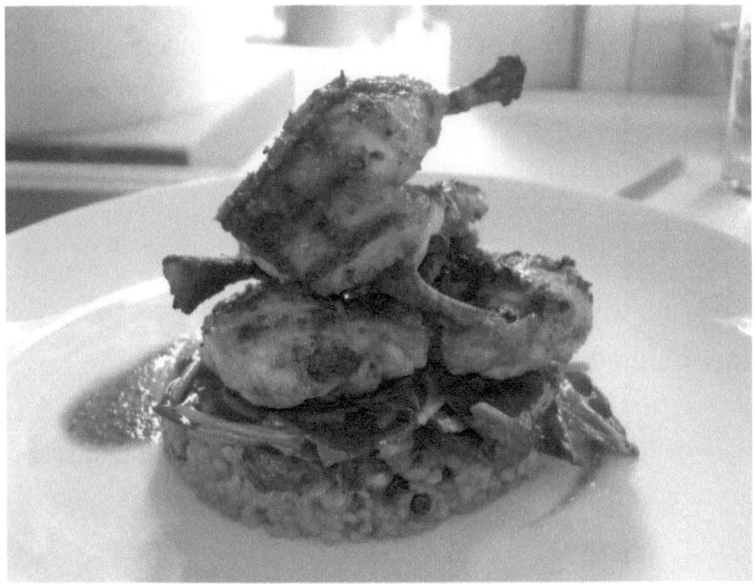

If you're looking for a fresh and delicious lunch recipe that doesn't require a lot of ingredients but will still fill you up, look no further than this low acid meal.

Yield: 2

Preparation Time: 45 minutes

List of Ingredients:

- 2 chicken breasts, boneless and skinless
- 1 Tbsp. olive oil + extra for greasing the grill
- 3 cups fresh baby spinach, trimmed and chopped
- Sea salt to taste

xxxxxxxxxxxxxxxxxxxxxxxxxxxxxxxxxxxx

Instructions:

Step 1: Thinly slice the chicken breasts. Set to the side for the moment.

Step 2: Preheat your grill to medium high heat. Lightly grease the grill's grate with olive oil.

Step 3: Brush one half of the chicken with olive oil. Sprinkle the sea salt over the area.

Step 4: Place the chicken on the grill and cook for about 5 to 10 minutes, or until the chicken is cooked completely through. Remove the cooked chicken from the grill and set on a plate. Cover the plate with foil to keep the chicken warm.

Step 5: Turn the heat up on the grill to high. Grease a piece of foil with olive oil.

Step 6: Place the baby spinach in the middle of the foil. Drizzle ½ Tbsp. of olive oil over the spinach and sprinkle with sea salt.

Step 7: Create a sealed pouch by folding the edges of the foil up and over the spinach. Place this pouch directly on the grill and cook for about 10 minutes.

Step: Carefully open the sealed pouch and dump the grilled spinach onto a serving plate. Place the cooked chicken from Step 4 directly on top of the spinach and serve while still warm.

Recipe 12: Winter Soup

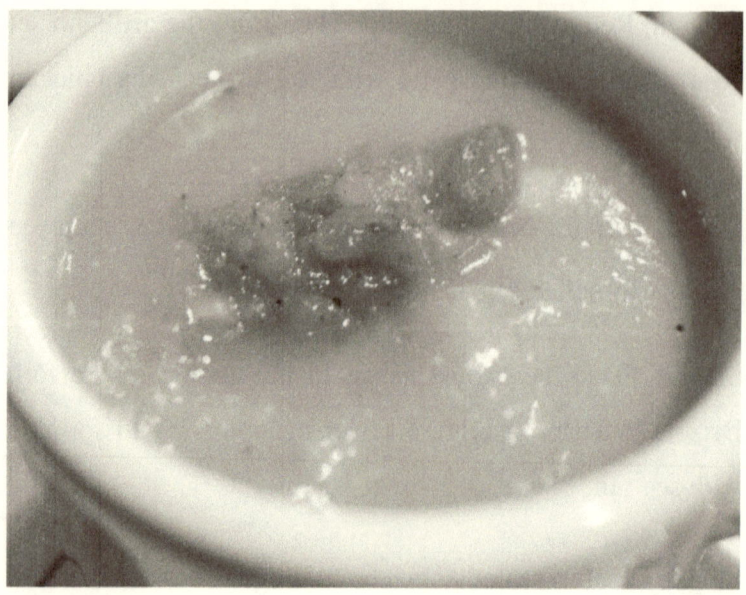

This roasted soup recipe features the delicious cool-season crop squash and makes a wonderful lunch for those cold fall and winter afternoons.

Yield: 2

Preparation Time: 1 hour 40 minutes

List of Ingredients:

- 1 winter squash seeded and halved
- 1 carrot, peeled and diced
- ½ celery stalk, chopped
- ¾ tsp. olive oil
- 2 cups vegetable broth, low-sodium
- Pinch cloves
- Pinch cumin
- Sea salt, to taste
- 2 Tbsp. plain yogurt, low-fat

xxxxxxxxxxxxxxxxxxxxxxxxxxxxxxxxxxxx

Instructions:

Step 1: Turn the oven to 350-degrees and allow to preheat for several minutes. Prepare a baking sheet by lining it with foil. Lay the halved winter squash onto the baking sheet with the cut side of the vegetable laying down. Roast the squash in the oven for about 50 to 55 minutes. Scoop out the pulp and place in a bowl. Set the bowl to the side for the moment.

Step 2: Pour the oil in a soup pan. Set the pan on the stove over medium heat and then add the celery and carrot. Cover the pan and let cook, making sure to stir occasionally, for about 10 minutes.

Step 3: Stir the cumin and cloves into the soup pan, and cook for another minute or two. Stir in the vegetable broth and the roasted squash. Let the mixture come to a boil before reducing the heat to low.

Step 4: Cover the soup pan and let simmer for 20 minutes. Remove the pan from heat and let cool slightly.

Step 5: Pour the soup into the blender and blend until smooth. For easier blending, do this in batches. Transfer the blended soup back into the pan and cook on medium high for another few minutes.

Step 6: Season the soup with salt to taste. Top the soup with yogurt before serving.

Recipe 13: Corn and Tomato Soup

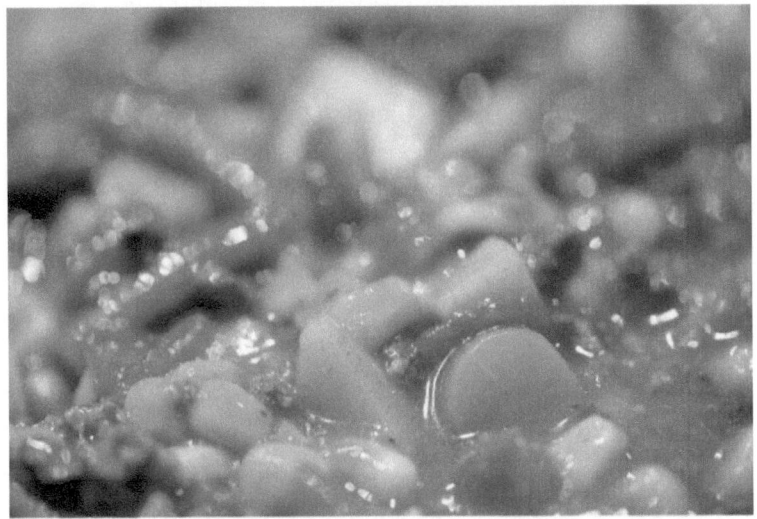

Feel your belly with this corn and tomato soup without agitating acid reflux symptoms.

Yield: 8

Preparation Time: 2 hours

List of Ingredients:

- 6 pounds tomatoes, seeded and cut into wedges
- 2 tsp. olive oil
- ½ cup white onion, diced
- 4 garlic cloves, minced
- 4 corn cobs
- 4 cups water
- 4 cups vegetable or chicken broth, low-sodium
- 1 cup of white wine
- 2 Tbsp. thyme
- 2 Tbsp. rosemary
- Spray olive oil

xxxxxxxxxxxxxxxxxxxxxxxxxxxxxxxxxxxx

Instructions:

Step 1: Preheat the oven to 400-degrees. Place the tomatoes on a roasting pan. Spray the tomatoes lightly with the spray olive oil. Place the tomatoes in the preheated oven and roast for 60 minutes.

Step 2: Place the corn cobs into a large pot. Fill with water until the cobs are covered and set on the stove. Turn the heat on high and let boil. Cook the corn cobs for about 10 minutes.

Step 3: Remove the corn cobs from the pot and let cool to touch. Cut the kernels from the cob. Set the corn kernels to the side for the moment.

Step 4: Pour the olive oil into a large pot. Place the pot on the stove over the medium heat. Add the onions and sauté until golden brown.

Step 5: Add the corn kernels and the garlic into the large pot. Cook for about 3 minutes before removing the pot from heat.

Step 6: Puree the roasted tomatoes in a blender until smooth. Transfer the pureed tomatoes into the pot. Add the remaining ingredients to the pot and stir.

Step 7: Place the pot on the stove and heat for about 20 minutes. Scoop the soup into serving bowls and serve while still warm.

Recipe 14: Roasted Broccoli

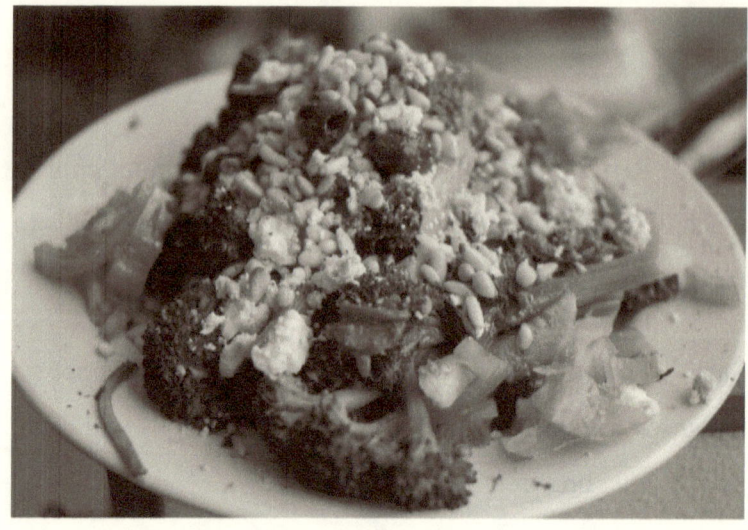

Roasted broccoli is a simple low acid meal that works well as a side for dinner or a small lunch.

Yield: 2

Preparation Time: 45 to 50 minutes

List of Ingredients:

- 3 cups ice water
- ½ pound fresh broccoli, cut into spears
- Olive oil cooking spray
- Pinch rosemary, dried and crushed
- Pinch sea salt

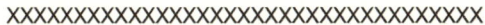

Instructions:

Step 1: Fill a pan with water. Place the pan on the stove over high heat and bring the water to a boil. Once boiling, place a steamer in the pan.

Step 2: Add the broccoli to the steamer basket and let cook for about 15 minutes.

Step 3: While the broccoli is cooking, pour the ice water into a large bowl. Set to the side for the moment.

Step 4: Remove the broccoli from the steamer. Immediately place the steamed broccoli into the bowl of ice water. Let the broccoli cool completely before draining the water off the vegetable.

Step 5: Preheat your oven to 400-degrees. Put a roasting pan in the preheated oven and let heat.

Step 6: Using oven mitts, carefully remove the heated pan from the oven and spray with the olive oil.

Step 7: Position the broccoli on the coated pan. Sprinkle the broccoli with the crushed rosemary and sea salt.

Step 8: Place the pan back in the oven and roasted for 20 minutes. Make sure to flip the broccoli every 5 minutes to ensure proper roasting on all sides.

Recipe 15: Low Acid Chicken Salad

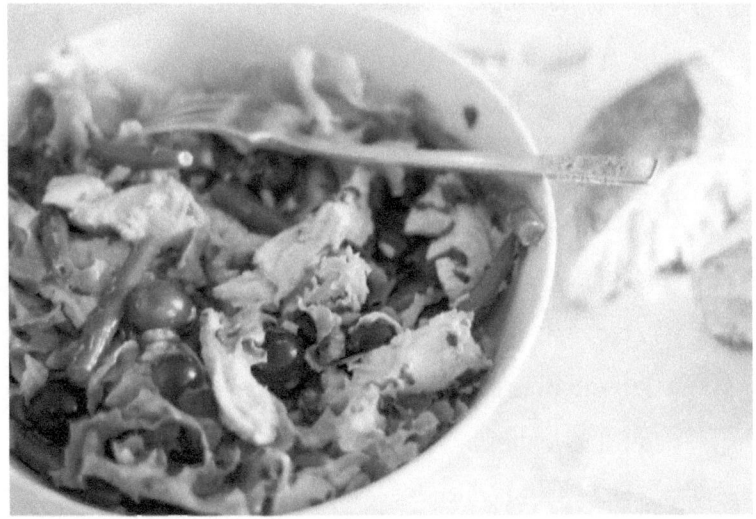

This traditional lunch meal is low in acid without giving up any tastes or flavors.

Yield: 8

Preparation Time: 50 minutes

List of Ingredients:

- 2 pounds chicken breast
- 1 cup white wine
- 8 cups water
- 4 garlic cloves, minced
- 8 celery ribs, diced
- 8 Tbsp. mayonnaise, reduced-fat
- ½ tsp. salt
- Ground black pepper, to taste
- Lettuce leaves

xxxxxxxxxxxxxxxxxxxxxxxxxxxxxxxxxxx

Instructions:

Step 1: In a large pot, mix the white wine and water together. Place the pot on the stove and bring the mixture to a boil.

Step 2: Reduce the heat a bit and add the chicken breasts. Let the chicken poach for 15 minutes. The inside of the chicken much reach an internal temperature of at least 160-degrees.

Step 3: Remove the pot from the stove and let the chicken cool to touch. Cut the cooled chicken into cubes. Transfer the cubed chicken to a large bowl. Cover the bowl and let the chicken chill in the fridge.

Step 4: Once the chicken has chilled, add the minced garlic, diced celery, mayonnaise, salt and black pepper. Mix until well combined.

Step 5: Spread the chicken salad over a large lettuce leaf. Roll the leaf up to make for easier consumption and serve immediately.

Chapter IV - Dinner Recipes for Acid Reflux

xxxxxxxxxxxxxxxxxxxxxxxxxxxxxxxxxxxxxx

Recipe 16: GERD-Friendly Chili

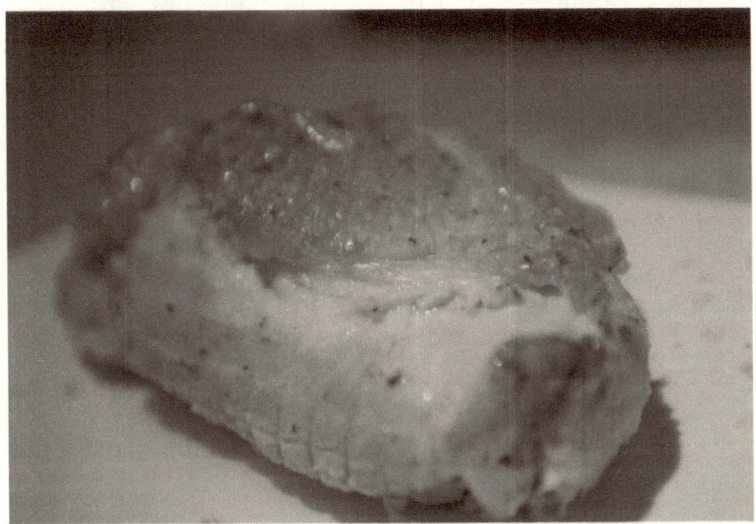

Chili is generally off limits to those suffering with acid reflux. This two bean turkey chili recipe, however, allows GERD-suffers to enjoy chili without causing problems.

Yield: 6

Preparation Time: 40 to 45 minutes

List of Ingredients:

- 1 15-ounce can bean, white or cannellini, rinsed and drained
- 4 cups cooked turkey breast, diced
- 1 14-ounce can chicken broth, reduced-sodium
- 2 cups corn
- 2 4-ounce cans roasted green chiles, diced
- 1 15-ounce can black beans, rinsed and drain
- 1 tsp. oregano
- 1 tsp. cumin (this ingredient can be eliminated if not tolerated)
- 1 tsp. garlic powder (this ingredient can be eliminated if not tolerated)
- ½ tsp. salt, kosher
- ¼ cup cilantro, chopped
- ½ cup sour cream, reduced-fat + more for garnish if desired
- Reduced fat shredded cheese, for garnish

xxxxxxxxxxxxxxxxxxxxxxxxxxxxxxxxxxxxx

Instructions:

Step 1: Pour ½ cup of the cannellini or white beans in a food processor. Add ¼ cup of chicken broth. Cover with the lead and pulse until the mixture is smooth.

Step 2: Transfer the bean puree mixture to a large pot and add the remaining chicken broth. Stir in the black beans, turkey, chiles, corn, oregano, cumin, salt and garlic powder.

Step 3: Turn the heat under the pot on medium high and bring the mixture to a boil. Once is reaches a boil, reduce heat and let simmer uncovered for about 25 minutes.

Step 4: Remove the pot from heat. Remove ¼ cup of the chili and pour into a mixing bowl. Add ½ cup of sour cream and stir until well combined. Add the cilantro and stir. Transfer this mixture back into the pot of chili and stir.

Step 5: Divide the chili between serving bowls and top with shredded cheese and sour cream.

Recipe 17: Bite-Sized Coconut Chicken

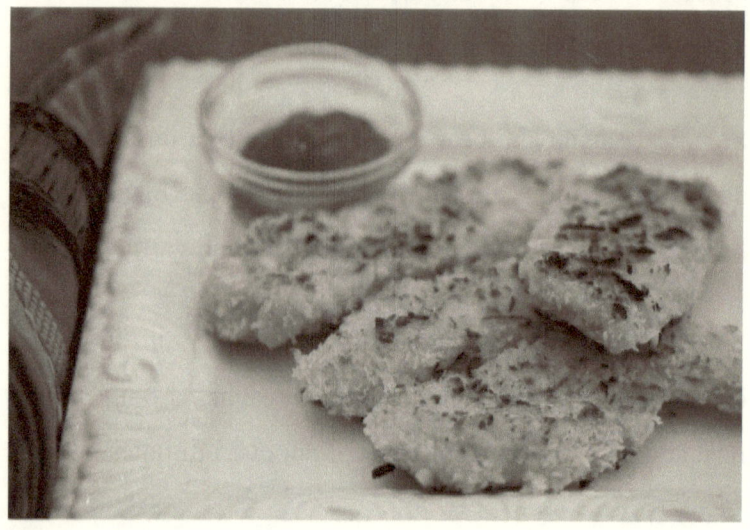

These delicious and non-acid reflux aggravating chicken bites will please all members of your family, no matter what their age.

Yield: 4

Preparation Time: 30 to 35 minutes

Chicken Ingredients:

- 1-pound chicken, skinless and boneless
- 3 large egg whites
- ½ tsp. garlic powder
- ¼ tsp. ginger
- 1 cup shredded coconut
- 1 tsp. sea salt
- Coconut oil

Coconut Glaze Ingredients:

- 1/3 cup coconut milk
- 1/3 cup raw honey
- ¼ cup shredded coconut
- ¼ tsp. ginger
- 1 Tbsp. lime juice
- Pinch sea salt
- Water

XXXXXXXXXXXXXXXXXXXXXXXXXXXXXXXXXX

Instructions:

Step 1: Turn the oven to 425-degrees and let preheat. Prepare a baking sheet by lining the bottom with parchment paper and then set the baking sheet aside for the moment.

Step 2: Start preparing the chicken bites by placing the 1 cup of shredded coconut into a shallow dish. Set the dish to the side for the moment.

Step 3: In a large mixing bowl, whisk the egg whites, salt, garlic and ginger for about 2 to 4 minutes. You want the mixture to be fluffy and light.

Step 4: Cut the skinless and boneless chicken into 1-inch bite-sized cubes. Place the chicken cubes into the egg white mixture and toss until completely coated.

Step 5: Next, completely coat the chicken cubes in the coconut flakes, before coating them again in the egg white mixture and a second time in the coconut flakes. This the coating process goes egg white mixture, coconut flakes, egg white mixture, coconut flakes.

Step 6: Lay the coated chicken cubes on the prepared baking sheet from Step 1. Lightly brush each top of the chicken cubes with coconut oil.

Step 7: Place the chicken cubes in the preheated oven and bake for about 5 minutes. Remove the baking sheet from the oven. Turn the chicken cubes over and brush the new tops with coconut oil.

Step 8: Place the chicken cubes back into the oven and bake for another 5 minutes. The coconut should be golden brown and the chicken cooked through completely.

Step 9: Make the coconut sauce by mixing the coconut milk, honey, ginger, lime juice, salt and ¼ cup shredded coconut together in a small pot. If necessary, add a little bit of water to the mixture at a time until you reach the desired consistency of the glaze.

Step 10: Place the small pot on the stove over medium heat. Bring the mixture to a simmer while stirring constantly. Remove from heat.

Step 11: Transfer the cooked chicken bites into a large mixing bowl. Pour the glaze from Step 10 immediately over the chicken bites. Toss until the chicken bites are completely coated.

Step 12: Serve the chicken bites while warm with a side of your favorite steamed vegetables.

Recipe 18: Salmon Patties and Homemade Tarter Herb Sauce

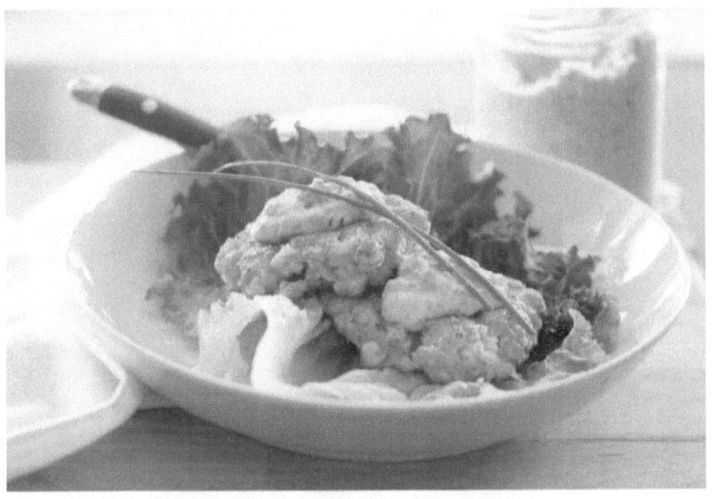

This low acid recipe is filled with protein and includes a delicious homemade tartar sauce.

Yield: 6

Preparation Time: 30 to 45 minutes

Salmon Patty Ingredients:

- 3 7½-ounce cans Alaskan pink salmon, drained
- 1 ½ cups breadcrumbs, divided
- ¼ cup parsley, chopped
- 2 Tbsp. celery, chopped
- 3 egg whites, lightly beaten
- ½ tsp. lemon peel, grated
- 1 tsp. seafood seasoning
- 2 Tbsp. olive oil, divided

Tartar Sauce Ingredients:

- ¼ cup plain yogurt, non-fat
- ¼ cup mayonnaise, reduced-fat
- ¼ cup relish
- ¼ tsp. seafood seasoning
- 1 tsp. ground mustard
- ½ tsp. tarragon

xxxxxxxxxxxxxxxxxxxxxxxxxxxxxxxxxxxx

Salmon Patty Instructions:

Step 1: Mix the salmon, parsley, celery, egg whites. Lemon peel, seafood seasoning and 1 cup of breadcrumbs together in a large bowl.

Step 2: Scoop 1/3 cup of the mixture from the bowl and form the mixture into a patty. Continue in this manner until you have used all the mixture and made 12 patties.

Step 3: Pour the remaining breadcrumbs into a shallow dish. Coat each patty with the breadcrumbs. Make sure to coat each side of the patties.

Step 4: In a skillet, add 1 Tbsp. of olive oil. Place the skillet on the stove and warm over medium heat.

Step 5: Sauté the patties in the skillet for about 12 minutes, making sure to turn once during the cooking process. You want the patties to be crisp and golden.

Herbed Tartar Sauce Instructions:

Step 1: Mix all the ingredients together in a mixing bowl until well combined. Place the bowl in the fridge and let chill for about 15 minutes.

Step 2: Serve the herbed tartar sauce with the salmon patties.

Recipe 19: Low Acid Grilled Korean Beef

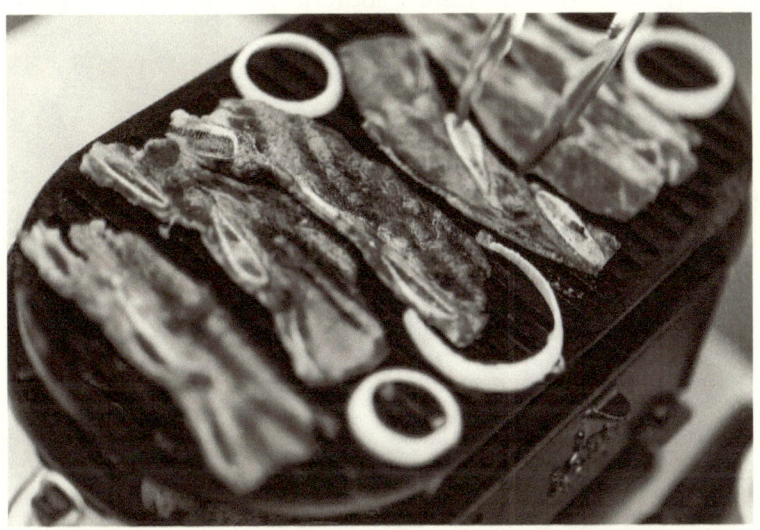

You won't have to worry about this oriental beef dish causing any problems with your acid reflux. So you can sit back and enjoy a delicious meal.

Yield: 4

Preparation Time: 3 hours to marinate + 30 to 45 for prep and cooking

List of Ingredients:

- 1-pound beef sirloin, sliced thinly
- ½ white or yellow onion, peeled and chopped Julienne-style
- 1 green onion, chopped
- 1 carrot, peeled and chopped Julienne-style
- 1 Tbsp. sesame oil
- 3 Tbsp. tamari
- 1 Tbsp. sesame seeds
- 1 garlic clove, peeled and minced
- 1 tsp. raw honey
- ½ tsp. sea salt

xxxxxxxxxxxxxxxxxxxxxxxxxxxxxxxxxxxx

Instructions:

Step 1: Mix the minced garlic, sesame oil, salt, honey and sesame seeds together in a container with a lid.

Step 2: Add the onions, carrots and green onions to the container. Add in the beef.

Step 3: Secure the lid in place and shake the container for several seconds until everything inside is mixed well. Place the container in the fridge and let chill for about 3 hours.

Step 4: Turn your outdoor grill to high heat.

Step 5: Drain the marinade from the beef and vegetables, and place them on a baking sheet covered with aluminum foil. Make a sealed packet by folding the foil over the meat and vegetables.

Step 6: Place the sealed packet on the preheated grill and cook for about 20 to 25 minutes.

Step 7: Remove the sealed packet from the grill carefully and lay on a protected surface, such as a cutting board. Open one end of the sealed packet and let the steam escape for about a minute.

Step 6: Carefully dump the meat and vegetables out of the sealed packet and onto a serving dish. Serve while still hot.

Recipe 20: Vegetable Bean Soup

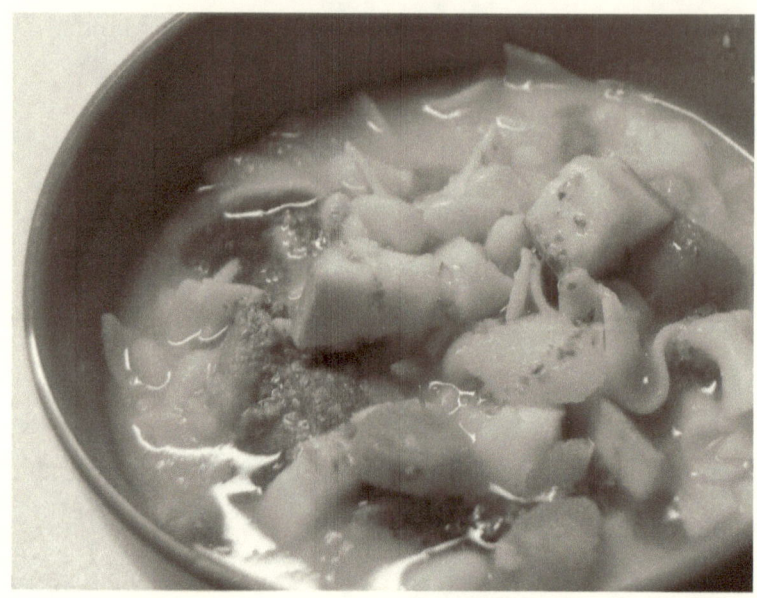

If you want a low acid meal that won't aggravate acid reflux but will fill you up and warm your body, look no further than this vegetable bean soup!

Yield: 6 to 8

Preparation Time: 2 hours 30 minutes

List of Ingredients:

- 16 cups water
- ½ cup kidney beans, dried
- 1/3 cup brown rice, long grain
- 2 tomatoes, stem removed and cut into wedges
- 1 onion, diced
- 1 tsp. oregano
- 1 tsp. basil
- 1 carrot, diced
- 2 sweet potatoes, skinned and diced
- 1 zucchini, skinned and diced
- ¼ pound cabbage, diced
- 1/8 tsp. celery seeds
- ¼ cup parsley, chopped
- ¼ tsp. marjoram

xxxxxxxxxxxxxxxxxxxxxxxxxxxxxxxxxxxx

Instructions:

Step 1: Pour 2 quarts of water into a large pot and place the pot on the stove and turn the heat on high. Place the beans in the pot and bring the water to a boil. Once the water boils, remove the pot from heat and let stand for 60 minutes.

Step 2: Drain the water from the beans.

Step 3: Add 3 cups of fresh water into the pot with the beans. Place the pot on the stove and cook for about 30 minutes.

Step 4: Add all the vegetables, except for the tomatoes and sweet potatoes, and all the seasonings. Stir together and let simmer for about 20 minutes.

Step 5: Add the sweet potatoes and tomatoes into the mixture and cook for an additional 30 minutes.

Step 6: Divide the soup between serving bowls and serve while still warm.

Chapter V - Dessert and Snack Recipes for Acid Reflux

xxxxxxxxxxxxxxxxxxxxxxxxxxxxxxxxxxx

Recipe 21: Low Acid Raspberry Cobbler

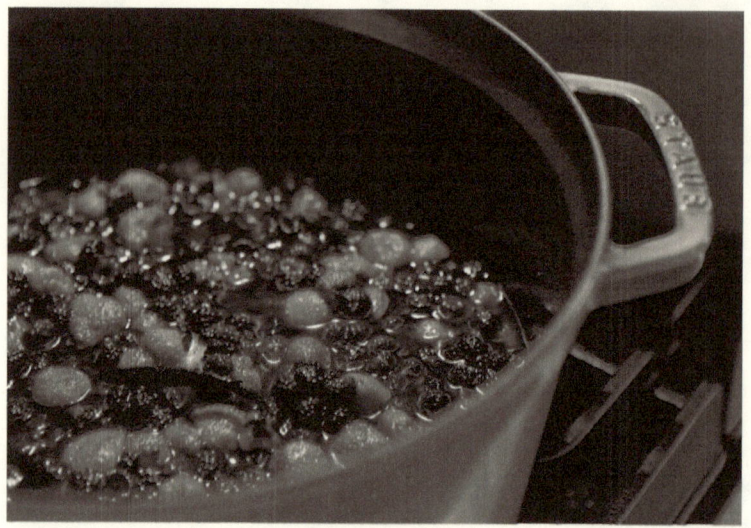

What's so great about this cobbler is that it is low in acid and cranberries, blueberries or blackberries can be used as a substitution for raspberry!

Yield: 8

Preparation Time: 1 hour 20 minutes

List of Ingredients:

- 1 cup granulated sugar
- 2 cups flour, all-purpose
- ½ tsp. salt
- 2 ½ tsp. baking powder
- 2/3 cup milk
- 3 Tbsp. unsalted butter, melted
- 1 large egg, lightly beaten
- 1 tsp. vanilla extract
- 2 cups raspberries

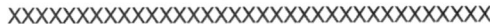

xxxxxxxxxxxxxxxxxxxxxxxxxxxxxxxxxxxx

Instructions:

Step 1: Preheat the oven to 350-degrees. Prepare a square baking pan by spraying the bottom and sides with cooking oil. Set the pan to the side for the moment.

Step 2: In a large mixing bowl, stir together the sugar, flour, salt and baking powder. Mix in the melted butter, vanilla, milk and beaten egg until well combined.

Step 3: Fold in the raspberries.

Step 4: Pour the batter into the prepared pan. Place the pan in the oven and bake for about 45 minutes. The top of cobbler should be firm and tight.

Step 5: Let the cobbler cool a bit before serving. If desired, add a scoop of vanilla ice cream to the top or side of the cobbler.

Recipe 22: I Can't Believe It's Not Fudge

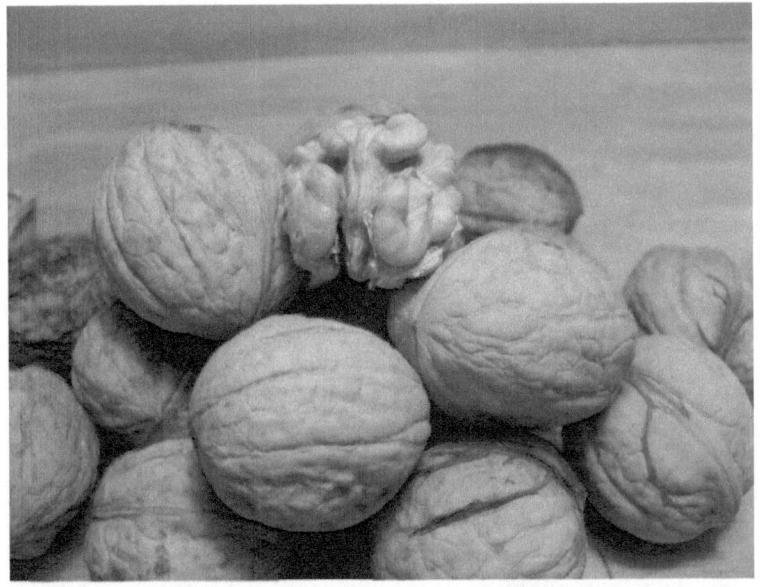

This fudge recipe doesn't contain the traditional ingredients that you expect but it's delicious nonetheless and won't aggravate acid reflux,

Yield: 8 to 10

Preparation Time: 2 hours 30 minutes

List of Ingredients:

- 1 cup dates, pitted
- 2 cups cashews, soaked and drained
- 2 Tbsp. carob powder
- 1 cup raisins
- 1 cup walnuts, chopped
- 1 cup flaxseed meal
- ½ cup water, distilled
- ½ cup pineapple juice

xxxxxxxxxxxxxxxxxxxxxxxxxxxxxxxxxxxxxx

Instructions:

Step 1: Blend together the dates, carob powder, cashews, raisins, walnuts and pineapple juice in a blender or food processor. Continue blending until smooth.

Step 2: Stir in the water and flaxseed meal until well combined.

Step 3: Press the mixture into a baking sheet. Place the sheet in the freezer for about 2 hours. Cut the fudge into squares before serving.

Recipe 23: Low Acid Almond Meringues

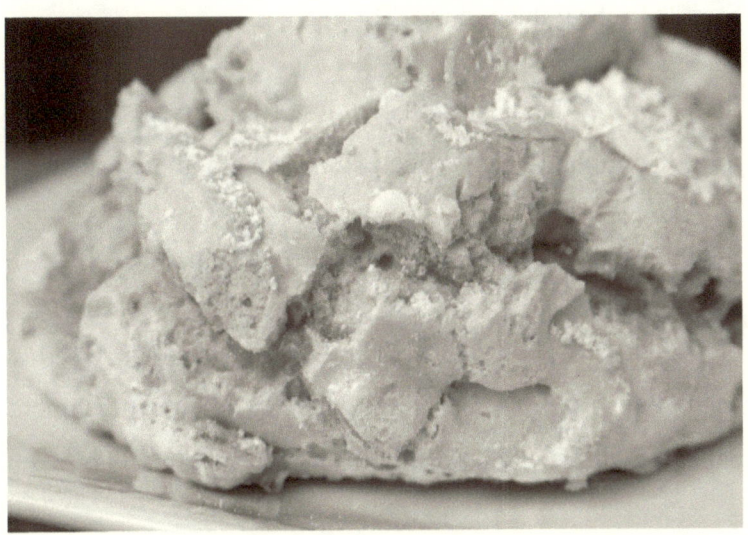

Requiring only 3 ingredients, these almond meringues won't annoy acid reflux symptoms.

Yield: 2 to 3

Preparation Time: 2 hours and 20 minutes

List of Ingredients:

- 3 large egg whites
- ¾ cup granulated sugar
- 1/3 cup sliced almonds, toasted and crushed

XXXXXXXXXXXXXXXXXXXXXXXXXXXXXXXXXXXXX

Instructions:

Step 1: Preheat the oven to 225-degrees.

Step 2: Beat the egg whites and salt until peaks begin to form. Continue to beat while adding the granulated sugar.

Step 3: Line a baking sheet with parchment paper.

Step 4: Transfer the meringues into a pastry bag. Use the pastry bag to pipe the meringues directly onto the parchment paper n a lattice style. Sprinkle the almonds directly on top.

Step 5: Place the baking sheet in the preheated oven and bake for about 60 minutes. You want the meringues to be a golden pale color with a crispy texture.

Step 6: Remove the baking sheet from the oven and let the meringues cool for about an hour before serving.

Recipe 24: Low Acid Angel Food Cake

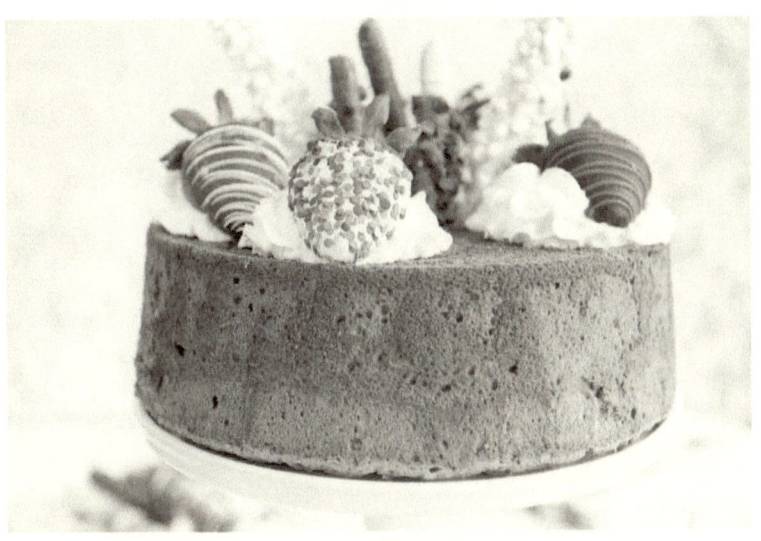

Another traditional dessert, this angel food cake recipe is low in acid, which means you can enjoy the treat even if you suffer from acid reflux.

Yield: 8

Preparation Time: 70 to 75 minutes

List of Ingredients:

- ¾ cup + ¼ cup granulated sugar
- 1 cup cake flour, sifted
- 1 tsp. cream of tartar
- ½ tsp. salt
- 12 large egg whites, room temperature
- 2 tsp. vanilla

xxxxxxxxxxxxxxxxxxxxxxxxxxxxxxxxxxxxx

Instructions:

Step 1: Preheat the oven to 375-degrees.

Step 2: Whisk together the flour and ¾ cup of sugar.

Step 3: In a second bowl, beat the egg whites until they are thick. Stir in the salt, cream of tartar and vanilla. Continue to beat until stiff peaks begin to form. Stir in the remaining ¼ cup of sugar.

Step 4: Combine the flour mixture to the egg mixture until well mixed. Pour this mixture into a non-stick tube pan. Place the pan in the oven and bake for about 30 to 35 minutes.

Step 5: Remove the pan from the oven and let cool before serving.

Recipe 25: Pound Cake

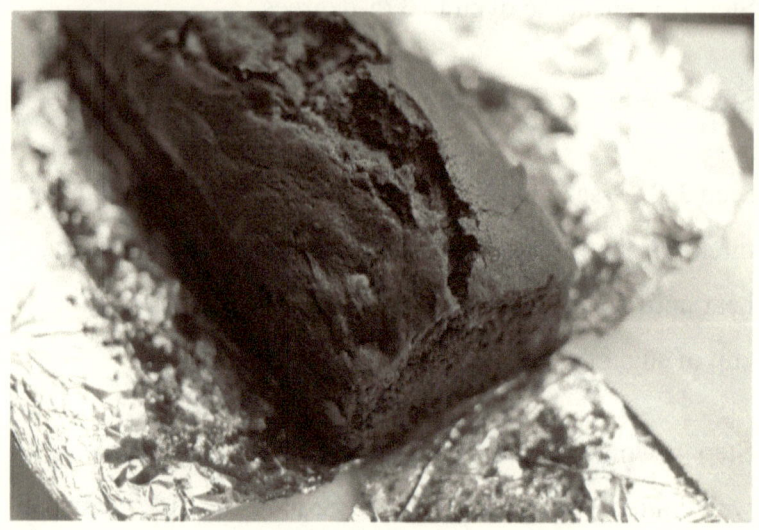

This traditional dessert is simple to make and won't cause any problems for acid reflux sufferers.

Yield: 6 to 8

Preparation Time: 75 to 80 minutes

List of Ingredients:

- 2 cups flour, all-purpose
- ¼ tsp. salt
- 1 Tbsp. baking powder
- 1 ½ cups granulated sugar
- ½ cup unsalted butter, softened
- 4 large egg whites, lightly beaten
- 2 tsp. vanilla extract
- 1 ½ cups sour cream, fat-free
- Powdered sugar, optional

xxxxxxxxxxxxxxxxxxxxxxxxxxxxxxxxxxxxx

Instructions:

Step 1: Preheat your oven to 350-degrees. Prepare a bundt pan by spraying the bottom and sides with cooking oil. Set the pan to the side for the moment.

Step 2: In a small bowl, shift together the flour, salt and baking soda. Set to the side for the moment.

Step 3: In a large mixing bowl, cream the butter and sugar together. Stir in the egg whites, vanilla and sour cream. Continue stirring until well mixed.

Step 4: Gradually stir the flour mixture into the butter mixture until combined but not over mixed.

Step 5: Transfer the batter into the prepared bundt pan from Step 1. Place the pan in the oven and let bake for about an hour. The pound cake is done when a toothpick inserted in the middle comes out clean.

Step 6: Remove the pan from the oven and let cool for completely before turning the cake out of the pan. Dust with powdered sugar before serving.

Chapter VI - Acid Reflux Tips and Considerations

xxxxxxxxxxxxxxxxxxxxxxxxxxxxxxxxxxxxx

While the recipes won't agitate acid reflux symptoms, they are in no way the only foods you can consume. But since the list of foods you can have is so extensive, I decided that it would be better to list the foods that you should avoid if suffering from acid reflux.

Foods to Avoid

- Spice, fatty and fried foods
- Citrus fruits and citrus juices
- Foods with a tomato base, such as pasta sauce, pizza and salsa
- Chocolate
- Garlic and onions
- Alcoholic beverages
- Caffeinated drinks
- Mint flavorings
- Tea and coffee (both decaffeinated and caffeinated)
- Carbonated drinks

Acid Reflux Triggers

Along with the above "foods to avoid", there are several non-food related things that can trigger acid reflux.

- Smoking – Studies have shown that smoking can contribute to GERD in many ways including increasing the acid secretion and damaging mucus membranes.
- Pregnancy – Many women develop acid reflux while they are pregnant. This is usually due to the increase in hormone levels and pressure caused by the growing fetus.
- Obese or Overweight – Carrying excessive weight is a common situation that leads to acid reflux. Losing the extra weight will go a long way to improving GERD symptoms.
- Eating before Bed – Consuming any size meal before going to bed is nothing more than an invitation inviting acid reflux symptoms to flare-up.
- Exercise – While exercising can temporarily aggravate acid reflux symptoms, that doesn't mean you should cut it out of your daily life. In fact,

increasing exercise can help reduce weight, thus preventing GERD.

About the Author

Heston Brown is an accomplished chef and successful e-book author from Palo Alto California. After studying cooking at The New England Culinary Institute, Heston stopped briefly in Chicago where he was offered head chef at some of the city's most prestigious restaurants. Brown decide that he missed the rolling hills and sunny weather of California and moved back to his home state to open up his own catering company and give private cooking classes.

Heston lives in California with his beautiful wife of 18 years and his two daughters who also have aspirations to follow in their father's footsteps and pursue careers in the culinary arts. Brown is well known for his delicious fish and chicken dishes and teaches these recipes as well as many others to his students.

When Heston gave up his successful chef position in Chicago and moved back to California, a friend suggested he use the internet to share his recipes with the world and so he did! To date, Heston Brown has written over 1000 e-books that contain recipes, cooking tips, business strategies for catering companies and a self-help book he wrote from personal experience.

He claims his wife has been his inspiration throughout many of his endeavours and continues to be his partner in business as well as life. His greatest joy is having all three women in his life in the kitchen with him cooking their favourite meal while his favourite jazz music plays in the background.

Author's Afterthoughts

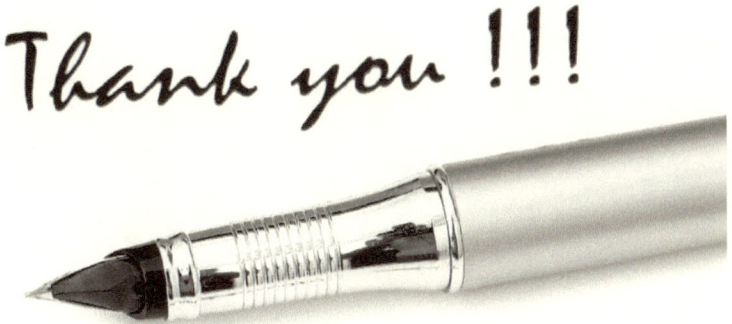

Thank you to all the readers who invested time and money into my book! I cherish every one of you and hope you took the same pleasure in reading it as I did in writing it.

Out of all of the books out there, you chose mine and for that I am truly grateful. It makes the effort worth it when I know my readers are enjoying my work from beginning to end.

Please take a few minutes to write an Amazon review so that others can benefit from your opinions and insight. Your review will help countless other readers make an informed choice

Thank you so much,

Heston Brown

www.ingramcontent.com/pod-product-compliance
Lightning Source LLC
Chambersburg PA
CBHW021228280526
45784CB00005B/2015